TYPE ONE DIABETES DOESN'T STOP ME

JORDYN M JONES

COPYRIGHT

Cover Portrait by: Morgan Jameson of Less is Morgan Photography

I dedicate this book to all people dealing with Type One Diabetes and the life burden that comes with it. I also dedicate this book to the family members and friends of those dealing with Type One Diabetes and the worry it brings onto them.

CONTENTS

INTRODUCTION

I wrote this book to raise awareness for Type One Diabetes. To make any donations please visit http://www.jdrf.org/ All donations are greatly appreciated, and every penny counts.

I was diagnosed with Type One Diabetes (T1D) in 2013 and have been battling a different way of life ever since. Everyone has their own story but here on these pages I am going to tell you mine. Thank you for taking the time to read my story. I hope to inform people of what having T1D means and how to offer support to those dealing with the chronic illness.

1

GROWING UP

I WAS BORN on August 13, 2000, into a spectacular family. We lived in the town of Alexandria, MN, with a population of a little over 10,000 people. I grew up as the youngest of four girls. My three older sisters have been my best friends since my first step on earth and will be until my last breath. Growing up on a gravel road with only a few neighbors incorporated an extended amount of family time in our household. My family and I got along extremely well. We always walked to the house of the gumball lady—a lady that kept a fully stocked gumball machine in her basement, or to the house of the licorice lady—a lady that always answered the door with a fresh piece of licorice in her hand. These were some of our favorite things to do, besides swimming in the 6,000 acres of Lake Miltona in our backyard. My life in Minnesota was a dream. It seemed like I was growing up with a perfect loving family, in a perfect grayish blue house, with a perfect plan for life.

If there is one thing I have learned it is that "plans" may not always turn out to be as perfect as we had hoped them to be. We can only live in the now. We cannot focus on the past or the future. Moving forward in the now, living day by day, is what makes us ready to deal with change and struggle as it comes at us.

On August 13, 2006, I had to say good-bye to my friends, and to the house in which I was born. Good-bye to the gravel roads on which I had learned to bike. Good-bye to the lake in which I had first learned to waterski at the age of four. Good-bye to the quiet neighborhood and the family fun. Good-bye to Minnesota. It was a good-bye to the old, and a hello to the new. 2006 was a year of a lot of change for my family, but change didn't seem all that bad. I learned that the way I reacted to change was the only thing I could control.

The new move to Green Bay unfortunately didn't come with the 6,000 acre Lake Miltona that we had left in Alexandria, but I embraced the change and the new house we lived in. As lovers of the water, my family and I immediately joined a water ski team in Wrightstown, WI about 30 minutes from our new home. This team eventually became a second family to me. Our love for the water turned into a passion for the sport. It brought new friendships and opportunities every day. The Waterboard Warriors ski team became my second home. The end of the summer of 2006 was my first summer of many more to come of practicing two days a week and performing two days a week to a crowd of people.

With a population that was ten times bigger than my previous "home" it was soon inevitable that I made more friends in Green Bay, Wisconsin. My gravel roads turned into paved streets, with sidewalks. My 6,000 acre lake turned into somewhat of a "pond." My empty neighborhood turned into neighborhoods and neighborhoods and more neighborhoods with people, people, and more people.

Shortly, my Mom noticed that I had the wonderful gift of jumping around like a monkey—I was strong and flexible. She decided to sign me up at a new gym opening up a short distance from my house. This was not just any gym, but a gymnastics gym, Air Force Gymnastics. I was the very first person to step foot into Air Force Gymnastics. As I took my first step into the clean, chalkless gym, little did I know I would continue to walk into that gym for the next 11 years. I soon learned that each day was a new attempt to get better, stronger, faster, and tougher.

2

_____

THE DIAGNOSIS

It was 2012 and we had lived in Green Bay for 6 years. I was 12 years old and my passion for gymnastics grew into something I could never have imagined. My coaches had pushed me harder than I ever thought possible. They gave me the confidence to follow my dreams. We spent a lot of time together and shared many special memories. The 16+ hours a week I spent at the gym included the absolute best and absolute worst moments of my life. My body was challenged in so many ways. I pushed past so many boundaries to become the strongest emotionally and physically I had ever been. Up to that point I was in level 7 and training to become a level 8 gymnast. I knew it would require even more from me emotionally and physically. I had already competed at many many meets, locally and statewide, but my mind was focused on one dream: college gymnastics. With a natural love and commitment for the sport, it was a realistic goal that felt like the culmination of what I had started as a little girl when I first discovered my passion for gymnastics.

———————

In January of 2013, I was given an opportunity to compete at a gymnastics meet in Texas. We could not say no to this opportunity. My sister Josie, my Mom, and I traveled to Dallas, Texas. When we arrived in Texas, we dropped our bags off at the hotel and I threw myself on the bed. I was so tired. I just wanted to go to sleep, and it was only 7:30 pm. I ended up dragging myself out of bed and going out to eat with my family at a little restaurant in our hotel. Oh the hunger. I remember being endlessly hungry that night. It was as if everything went straight through me. My Mom even noticed I drank three giant glasses of chocolate milk with my dish of pasta for dinner. Going to sleep that night I felt restless, and I woke up multiple times to use the bathroom. This should have felt unusual for me. However, this had been happening for as long as I could remember, and felt normal.

The next morning, I was very drowsy. The three of us went to an amusement fair. Josie had a love for sweets, and so, of course, we had to get some cotton candy. I wasn't in the mood for it and it gave me a terrible headache. That night I just wanted to stay in the hotel and rest, but Mom and Josie said we had to do something fun because we were in Texas. So, we decided to go to a rodeo. As we sat in the stands watching the rodeo, I noticed my mind drifting and suddenly all I could think of was my extreme tiredness and thirst once again. I thought, "When would it stop? Was this normal?" I had become quite irritable with people, and especially to my Mom. I didn't want to feel so terrible or talk to my Mom that way. I didn't understand why I was feeling the way I was.

The following morning I woke up and was ready to compete. I competed in all four events (Vault, Bars, Beam, Floor). Though most of the morning was a blur, the balance beam that day was one event I will never forget. I was warming up and felt cold, shaky, mentally foggy, and drowsy. As I got up to compete, I didn't feel confident, but it was time to give it my all. I was making it through my routine when my hands tried to make their way to the the beam during my back-handspring. I couldn't see well and I was getting dizzy. My hands went off center and I fell. I couldn't even find enough energy to be mad at myself. All I could think was that maybe I wasn't meant for this sport. Doubts crossed my mind about my dream for college gymnastics. At awards I received two medals. Each time I went up to receive an award I found myself so tired that it was hard to be happy. I hoped the feeling would go away when I got back to Green Bay.

We headed to the airport right after the gymnastics competition. Before boarding the plane I drank two big bottles of sprite. Once boarded, I immediately drank the water bottle my Mom gave me to save for the ride. We sat in our seats waiting for the flight attendants to announce the safety and take off rules. As soon as the flight attendant began to talk I instantly needed to use to bathroom. I used it two more times before we even took off! I was unaware of the ridiculousness of this, but my Mom wasn't.

I didn't know it at the time, but my Mom noticed my unusual behavior during our weekend trip in Texas. She noticed my unending thirst and unsatisfied hunger. The other things she may or may not have noticed, or that I had not even payed attention to, was my intermittent blurred vision, constant need to go to the bathroom, and extreme fatigue. Slowly, something unknown, was draining my confidence, straining my relationships, and changing my personality. What was this? What could be this detrimental to have so many effects to all aspects of my life? As I look back, I can see how unaware I was of the serious nature of my symptoms. I am truly grateful that my Mom paid attention to what was happening to me, because it ultimately saved my life.

It was the week that we came back from the the trip that completely changed my life as I knew it. My Mom brought me to the doctor to get some tests done. I sat in the waiting room with her for what felt like an hour -but was probably only a few minutes. I could clearly see the concern on my Mom's face while we waited for the nurse to call us back. Finally, they called my name and I followed the nurse to get my height and weight. At twelve years old I only weighed 70 pounds, and was not within a healthy range of height and weight. Once again a look of concern on my Mom's face told me something was wrong.

My doctor examined me and noticed the change in my body and how I hardly had any fat anywhere. She ordered a couple of tests. When she came back to give us the results, she talked in a slightly lower tone. She stated, "Her blood sugar...is unfortunately over 500 and she is suffering with Type One Diabetes." I looked at my Mom to see her reaction. At the age of twelve, I didn't know what Type One Diabetes was. I was laying on the exam table, weak and uncertain of what was happening to me, and I watched as the expression on my Mom's face changed from contentment to devastation. January 28, 2013, was the day I was diagnosed with Type One Diabetes.

My Mom is the strongest woman I know. When I saw the worried look in her eyes, I was filled with worry, too. Since I had had the same doctor for several years, we knew each other quite well. She gave me a hug as I walked out of the office that day, and it gave me strength for the tasks that would come in the next weeks, months, and even years.

Immediately after the visit my Mom and I picked up the insulin pens, the testing meter, the strips, the "shot" teddy bear, and packets of information. We were embarking on a journey to learn a lot more about that little organ called the pancreas.

DEFINING TYPE ONE DIABETES

For a moment I am going to step aside from my story and describe what Type One Diabetes is for those of you that are unaware. Type one diabetes is an autoimmune disorder. The cause is not known with certainty; however, I have been told by doctors it is most likely a virus attacking the pancreas that causes it to slowly stop working until it completely shuts off forever. This means the body is unable to produce the hormone insulin to break down sugars in the blood. As of right now, there are no preventative methods, and the pancreas will never be able to produce its own insulin again. This can happen to anyone at any time, though it is most common in children, which is why it is also called Juvenile Diabetes. It can lead to dangerous hyper-glycemia without proper treatment; however with the necessary insulin injections or pump therapy it can lead to severe hypoglycemia as well. For this reason, it is important to watch blood sugar levels closely and check in with doctors every few months to make sure dosages are correct.

If you or someone you know is dealing with symptoms of extreme thirst, extreme fatigue, blurred vision, frequent urination, interrupted sleep, and weight loss; it may be signs of Type One Diabetes.

There are actually two types of diabetes. Type One Diabetes and Type Two Diabetes are completely different diseases. The similar name can be deceiving to people, but for each type there are different challenges and treatment. In the end of this book I give more information on Type One Diabetes and the common misconceptions of it. Please refer to this section for more information about how you can help someone living with T1D.

LEARNING CURVE

On the car ride home from the doctor's office that day in January of 2013, I remember asking my mom, " When will this go away? When will I be normal again?" Her response was at first silent, and with that silence I began to feel tears roll down my face as I looked out the window trying to hide my sadness and confusion.

We got home and my Mom prepared my lunch and looked up carb counts online, while I was trying to understand how I was going to get over my fear of needles. I grabbed my blood sugar meter and pricked my own finger for the first time. The needle pierced my soft skin. Ouch! After a few days of a dozen pricks per day my skin toughened up and I became brave enough to do it myself.

Nothing scared me more than the moment my Mom said, "Okay honey, it is time to take your shot for lunch." I laid down on the couch and tried to find a place where I had at least a pinch of fat. Undiagnosed, my Type One Diabetes had made me lose so much weight that it made this very challenging. Even though my belly had no fat to pinch my mom found a way to get just enough for the tiny needle to go in. She counted to three and stuck it in. I immediately felt a cold sting and a little burn for about 10 seconds. I began to cry at the thought of having to go through this for the rest of my life.

After about a week of learning how to take care of myself and slowly getting back to a healthy weight, it was time to return to school. I was an extremely shy sixth grade girl, which did not make this process easy. I knew I would have to answer questions and explain what happened to me during that week of school I had missed. That was terrifying to think about. The day I came back and walked into homeroom, I found a pile of letters from my fellow classmates. On the letters they wrote stuff like "get better soon" and "we missed you." Even though "get better soon" didn't seem possible in that moment it warmed my heart and reminded me I wasn't alone.

My best friend at the time was one of the reasons I did not feel completely hopeless and devastated from my diagnosis. To this day, I cannot thank her enough for bringing me out of that low point in my life. I hung out with her quite often. Not once did she ask me to explain what was wrong with me, which allowed me to escape my diabetes and feel "normal" again. She looked out for me and told me when I did not look right, but she never gave me that "I feel bad for you" look, and I appreciated that. So often when people found out I had diabetes they felt bad for me and treated me like I was contagious or fragile in some way. If anything, that just made me feel singled out and alone. I hated feeling like I was the center of attention. For this I cannot say enough how thankful I am to my best friend. She never doubted my abilities, and never made me feel like a "lesser" version of myself. Even though I was extremely shy, our friendship gave me the confidence to be more open about my diabetes. It showed me first, that yes, I had Type One Diabetes and nothing is going to make it go away, and secondly, that it was not going to stop me from being me.

5

FIGHTING ASSUMPTIONS

The next few weeks at school, I was overwhelmingly asked by teachers and classmates what I was "allowed" to eat, and so on. Nothing bothered me more than the assumption that I was restricted on my diet. I didn't know how to explain this to people. I needed to learn how to stand up for myself. It bothered me because they really didn't understand what I was going through, and most didn't know anything about Type One Diabetes.

One day a teacher was bringing in candy for everyone and asked me what she could bring for me instead. When I told her I CAN eat candy she doubted me, and after this I knew I would run into people who didn't understand Type One Diabetes for the rest of my life. This is the very reason I gained the confidence to stand up for myself and tell people when their assumptions were wrong. Standing up for myself has helped me to raise awareness in a small but effective way to my circle of friends and family.

Two weeks after my diagnosis I was allowed to return to gymnastics. I knew gymnastics would challenge me to manage my diabetes, but since it was a huge part of my life I knew I had to find a way to make it work. I practiced about 16+ hours a week with hardly any days off all year round. Previous to my diagnosis, I had extreme fatigue at practice, due to high blood sugars. Returning with more normal sugars was incredibly energizing; however the hourly blood sugar checks, and constant fears of being too high or too low was a huge responsibility. I was not ready to take on all this responsibility at only 12 years old, but I had to if I wanted to continue the sport I loved.

Many nights during the first year of my diagnosis I would come home from gymnastics in tears because I felt so different than everyone else. It was taking up time in my practices to check my blood sugars so often and to sit out when I was too low or high. I would think about having to manage my sugars like this for the rest of my life and it was wearing me out. It seemed so devastating, but something inside of me wasn't going to give up.

My coaches became aware of my high and low blood sugar symptoms so they could keep an eye out for me. Since I did not have a continuous glucose monitoring device yet, during each 4.5 hour practice I would have to prick my finger and check up to 10 times. Four days a week of this became extremely exhausting, on top of the energy exhaustion from going to school and practice itself. This is when I reminded myself of the promise I had made upon my diagnosis. I had promised myself that I would never let Type One Diabetes stop me from achieving my dreams. And so I persevered.

6

"GRACIE"

My life changed in the month of May, in 2013. I had been managing my sugars and finding correct doses long enough that I was able to train and get my own insulin pump! At first I didn't know what it all meant besides the fact that I wasn't going to have to take injections anymore.

After a few trips down to the Children's Hospital to learn more about the pump I was convinced this would be the best thing that ever happened to me. When it was finally the day to pick the brand for my new pump, I had to learn all about the different options. There was so many options: pink, gray, or blue and Medtronic, Omnipop, or T-slim. It took me awhile to decide but I ended up picking a pink Medtronic Minimed. It gave me a little stress thinking about what I was going to do with the pump during my long gymnastics practices and ski practices each week. I flipped around too much for it to stay attached during gymnastics and it was not waterproof to wear skiing. I knew I would have to go through another learning curve with the doses. Despite that, I knew this was a better solution and would help me to manage my diabetes better.

Wow! Even though having a pump still meant changing infusion sites every three days and reloading with insulin, it was a huge improvement to the quality of my life. Once I got through the learning process, I was free to act more like a "normal" teenager.

I no longer had to go to the office every day at lunch to take a shot. Instead I could pull out my new little pink pancreas, and independently take my own insulin. My friends, who claimed to be the aunties of my pump, named her "Gracie." Gracie and I had a beautiful five year journey ahead of us.

7

PERSEVERANCE

THE PERSEVERANCE I had been developing since my diagnosis soon helped me to achieve one of my lifetime goals. It was still 2013 and it was time to start indoor water ski practices. It was like the first day coming back to school after my diagnosis all over again. I had to re-explain and re-correct all of the misconceptions regarding Type One Diabetes to my fellow teammates and coaches. However, this year I was so excited to start practicing "Doubles" with my partner that it didn't bother me as much answering the same questions over and over again. The more I could tell the facts of T1D to people I knew, the more it would continue to spread and help with awareness.

A few months before the summer of 2013 my doubles partner and I had to decide if we were going to compete at the Wisconsin State Waterski Tournament in the Doubles Competition. This is when two people perform acrobatically while on the water. We decided to give it a try. We had competed a couple times before, but now we were both stronger and had more years of experience.

June came faster than we had expected and it was time to hit the water. We practiced almost every night on land and water. I had to prepare a dance for the dock beforehand and think of a "theme" for our performance. My Mom was in charge of making my costume. It was only a five minute performance but we had to fit as much as we could in those five minutes without falling in order to place well.

Just like that it was July, and it was the night before the competition. A bunch of my ski team friends slept over and we all worked on my dance and got excited together! The next morning we woke up around five am to travel to Wisconsin Rapids. On the way down my Mom finished hand-sewing my costume and I got my hair and makeup done by my sisters and ski team friends. I trusted them and had no care in the world what I looked like. Most likely I knew it would be "extra" and very waterski style extreme makeup since the judges were seated far away. After I was all done getting ready, we just had to wait, wait, wait.

This whole time I saw my blood sugar rising from my adrenaline and had to do my best to keep it down. I needed to be in the right range in order to have my full strength and concentration to compete, so I watched my sugars very closely.

It was finally our turn, and my partner grabbed his skis and we walked out to the dock. We set up the rope on the dock and gave the nod to the judges that we were ready. As they announced our names I felt waves of nervousness and happiness rush through me all at once.

We skied the best we could have done, and that was that. We took third place and were headed to Nationals. I couldn't believe it, we had done it! Never once before had we placed at the State Tournament. We took our trophy home that night and started preparing for Nationals. We had to increase difficulty, become more precise, and more confident in only a few weeks.

Sooner than we had imagined, it was already August and it was time for Nationals. The last few weeks we had put in many hours of practice before and after team practices and increased the level of difficulty. The night before the competition we prepared and got any last minute details figured out.

The morning of Nationals we drove down to Janesville, WI with my friends and family. The same process of managing my blood sugars before we competed and getting my nerves out happened again. Finally, it was our time. We set up on the dock and once again waited for them to announce our names. The music started and we began.

The whole time we were competing, I couldn't help but think about the amazing opportunity it was. We had worked so hard for everything and as we landed on the beach I knew we nailed it. Our scores were remarkably higher than state. Our hard work had paid off.

We waited for results, and found out we took first place! It felt like a dream. I smiled for the rest of the night. I wasn't smiling at the fact that we were the best in the Nation but at the fact that our determination led us to that moment. This was my first boost of confidence that my Type One Diabetes wasn't going to stop me.

8

TEENAGE YEARS

In September of 2013, I started 7th grade. At the beginning of the year my science teacher had asked me if I wanted to do a presentation about Type One Diabetes. At first, I was extremely against the idea because of my shyness; however I ended up doing the presentation because I wanted to help people understand what the disease was. Even though there were only 15 people in my class that day, I know it has branched out to even more people since.

At the age of 13 I began to grow and gain weight. I realized my blood sugars varied more often and so did the amount of things that could affect them: days off of gymnastics versus days on, weather, stress, adrenaline, activity, and many more. I did not understand how all these things could have such an effect on my blood sugar levels. This meant many doctor phone calls and appointments to change dosages often. I found myself learning when and mathematically how to change these dosages myself. I become aware of how each factor would affect my blood sugar and estimated changes in doses each day based on that. It felt like an enormous task, but the responsibility of managing this made me mature and grow up a little faster than the average 13 year old girl may wish to.

With this enormous amount of pressure at such a young age, I developed some severe anxiety and depression. Many people with Type One Diabetes deal with mental health issues, but I didn't know this at the time. I thought maybe it was my fault and that I was complaining about things too much. For a few months I went to therapy for the anxiety I was dealing with. Even though I didn't want to keep going it slowly started to change my life. I had to ask myself, "Will I need therapy forever? How am I going to overcome this depression and anxiety?" Dealing with a chronic illness such as Type One Diabetes is a huge burden to carry. I knew I would face struggles for the rest of my life and deal with it the best I could, but realizing I was not alone helped me to face it. On the day of my last therapy appointment I felt confident and hopeful that I had made it through what seemed to be the hardest time of my life. Any time I have a bad day I think back to my therapist and the advice she gave me. From this experience I learned that it was important to seek help when I needed it.

9

CHALLENGES

In the summer of 2014 I was still trying to figure out how to use my insulin pump on the water while water skiing. I had grown, and I was more active in the summertime. This meant that I had to change all my insulin rates once again.

At ski practice if I was disconnected from my pump for too long it was dangerous because then I didn't get the 24 hour rates the pump was programmed to give me; but if I took too much insulin then I had low blood sugars which meant sitting out during practice to recover. I had to patiently wait for the blood glucose number to rise. Sadly, the pump was not waterproof so I couldn't risk wearing it while skiing. That summer was once again full of trial and error for me with my insulin pump, but by July and August I had it figured out. I would go to my morning gymnastics practices from 7:30 am - 12:00 pm and only connect back to my pump once every hour. Then, I would go to ski practice from 5:30 pm - 8:00 pm and connect to my pump about every hour there too. Well, I at least had it figured out for those couple of months. When fall came, and school started, and the weather changed, and I kept growing—it was trial and error all over again.

At this point in my life I still remembered what life without Type One Diabetes was like, and boy did I miss it. I wished that I could go back to a day when I could simply enjoy eating without worrying about the number of carbs it had, how much insulin I needed to take, and the fear of taking too much or too little insulin. I would have done anything to go back to the "normal" life I used to have. I missed it so much.

The summer of 2014 taught me one unforgettable lesson about my safety. I was with my family on our summer weekly boat trip, in Sturgeon Bay. Each year around my birthday we would travel up there and spend a week living and sleeping on our boat. Since my family was so close, it didn't bother us to be sleeping 7 people when there was only two beds available. One night, we were all cooking dinner in the cabin below when suddenly my legs gave out below me and I dropped to the floor. My face was pale as snow. I felt like I had no energy to pick myself up and move. One of my sisters raced to grab my blood sugar meter and checked me immediately. I was below 40 so it couldn't even read a number. Someone threw a root beer at me and I chugged the whole thing. Of course, it takes time for my blood sugar to rise up again. I laid there on the floor thinking that if I hadn't been with someone that knew I had Type One Diabetes, I could have been in a very dangerous situation. I was lucky to be with my family, or I could have died. I am thankful for this experience, because it taught me that I needed to wear a medical alert bracelet. My Mom and I went to the children's hospital and looked at the gift shop with all the stylish T1D bracelets they had. I was thankful for my Mom's keen sense of style, because she understood I had to get a couple different ones to match ALL my outfits. After all, I am a teenage girl. I may have Type One Diabetes, but my medical alert bracelet can still be pretty!

Ever since that day my Mom has asked me everyday, "Are you wearing your bracelet today?" I used to respond with a teenage eye roll and get annoyed by the comment, but now I am grateful for it. I realized a medical alert bracelet has the power to save my life.

10

THE START OF HIGH SCHOOL

It was 2015, and I was a freshman in high school. Going from a class of 18 at a small private school to a class of over 400 at a public school with almost 2,000 students was a big change, and quite stressful for me. There were so many new people to meet, and I was a very shy girl. Of course the first thing I was worried about was having to explain my Type One Diabetes to a whole new group of friends. I feared that I wouldn't fit in.

Each day I met a few new people and each time someone would ask me what that pink thing was at my hip. I had a bad habit of saying "it's an insulin pump" and then changing the subject for fear of what they might ask next. Even when I told people I had Type One Diabetes I found it incredibly difficult to accept the amount of people who didn't even know what it was. At first they would give me a confused look. How could I have diabetes and weigh only 90 lbs? They would be confused why I was on an insulin pump, as if that made it a more severe kind of diabetes. I didn't have the confidence to help them understand what Type One Diabetes was, but I tried my best.

I had a difficult time to look past people that judged me by the first thing they saw or heard. I walked around the halls every day and wore my pink pump, slightly hidden if possible because I was still afraid what people would think. All I hoped was that I would gain confidence to stand up for myself, and be able to help inform people about the truth of what it meant to live with Type One Diabetes.

11

OPPORTUNITIES

ABOUT A MONTH into my freshman year, I was given an amazing opportunity that would eventually give me more confidence than I had ever had before. I was contacted by some representatives of The Juvenile Diabetes Research Foundation to be the "spotlight"—standing on the stage at the Gala while a video played my story—of the upcoming Gala. I knew this meant all attention would be placed on me to tell my story in the form of a video, and I immediately told my Mom "no." If anything was more terrifying than giving myself shots it was the thought of being the center of attention in front of hundreds of people! We talked about it for a few weeks and I was persistent on not doing it. Eventually, she made me do it.

The first task was to do an interview on the radio explaining the gala and a little bit about myself. Next, filmmakers made a video featuring my life and how I managed my diabetes. They highlighted the burdens of having Type One

Diabetes, and the determination I have to not let it stop me from living my life. They filmed me doing gymnastics and they asked me a lot of questions about how we count carbs while preparing a meal. When I got the email that the video had been finished I was so excited to see it but also nervous because I had never been filmed like that before.

About a week before the Gala I watched the video about a dozen times. I was trying to imagine what it would feel like to stand up in front of the audience after it played. I later found out that nothing I imagined came close to the actual moment itself.

On the night of the Gala, my family and I arrived early so we could meet the celebrity of the night, James Jones. We sat and ate our food and listened to the auction. Waiting, waiting, waiting, and waiting, nervously of course for the video to play.

Finally, the time had come. The live auction was completed and a representative announced that we were about to watch the Fund a Cure video of the year. It started. While it was playing I gazed around the audience, my heart was racing. I watched my family at first and noticed their tears, but then I was surprised to look at the table next to them and there were more tears. And then I looked at the table next to them, and they had tears in their eyes, too. It was a whole room full of tears.

When the video had finished, I walked up to the front of the stage with the little boy who was spotlighted in the video with me and instantly the whole room stood up and clapped. I couldn't believe it. In that exact moment, something had changed in me. To see how many people were emotionally inspired by the video is something I will remember for the rest of my life. Around $400,000 was raised for research that night, and to say I was able to help fundraise that money is incredible. Sometimes thinking back to that night brings a few tears to my eyes even now, happy tears. I will always be so grateful that my Mom made me do this. It is still one of the most memorable days of my life.

12

A LIVING DREAM

After the JDRF Gala, my freshman year continued to get better and better. I was beginning to get very serious in my gymnastics career. After a previous year of injuries, this had to be my comeback year. Level 9 was a new level of intensity and I was developing skills that were considered dangerous because the risk of injury was high. Every day I had to walk in to practice fully energized and with my mental state fully attuned. This of course meant that managing my blood sugar levels was even more important than before. I learned that keeping a routine made it easiest to manage. I would eat similar snacks before practice, and I had to make sure to eat something during our 15 minute break. Our practices were 4.5 hours long. With my heavy school load, managing my diabetes, and practicing so much it was a busy and stressful time.

In March, it was time to compete against all the other Level 9 Gymnasts in the Wisconsin State Tournament. I competed the best I could have done at the time and ended with an all around score of 35.9. This was enough to qualify for Regionals. Regionals was the next step before Nationals. It was an extremely competitive and important meet. It was the only chance I had to qualify for Nationals, which I had never done before.

The preparation for Regionals began with increasing reps, increasing intensity, and increasing confidence. Since Regionals was located in Missouri, we drove down a few days before the competition so we could explore the city. Regionals had taken place in Missouri a few years earlier so it was fun to relive the experience again and visit the famous Gateway Arch in St. Louis one more time.

The day of competition came and I was ready. I knew all my hard work had paid off when I received a personal best all-around score of 36.3. I couldn't believe it! I had placed second and qualified for the Level 9 Western Nationals. I knew in the next few weeks I would have to get even better and stronger. Repetitions, repetitions, repetitions. Perfection, perfection, perfection. I put in more hours, more concentration, and pushed myself farther than I ever thought was possible.

Western Nationals was taking place in Missoula, Montana so we flew down a few days early and met up with some of my distant cousins. The next day we hiked up the "M" Mountain and toured the college campus. I was thinking about the competition the whole time, and still in amazement that I was going to compete the next day.

Finally, the day of the competition arrived. I was competing against the best gymnasts in the western nation, most of who had plans for college and elite gymnastics in their future. Sometimes I doubted myself and my abilities because of my diabetes. I hadn't heard of many T1D athletes that had made it to the top. This is because having Type One Diabetes and managing it with a sport was very challenging. On this day, I had to push those thoughts aside, and instead think of the hard work I had put into preparing for that day and the confidence I had developed along the way. I wanted to become a gymnast with Type One Diabetes that rose above the "normal" to do something unheard of and extraordinary.

I put on my Region Four leotard—maroon and black with a sparkly number four on the top—and the warmups they had given us upon arrival. It was time to start the competition. Beam was first, and all I had was a minute to prove myself. I had to show everything I had been working on for hours and hours in the past weeks. I stuck it, didn't fall, and felt confident throughout the routine. Next was floor, which I was most excited for because in my floor routine I could show my personality and skill all at once. As I was running towards my last tumbling pass I knew I had nailed it. I gave it my all and put all my emotion out there. Next was vault, which I had been struggling with the past few weeks, but I was ready to look past that and be happy with however it went. Finally, it was time for bars, my personal favorite. My hands had rips all over from the training the last few weeks. Rips are the gymnastics term for calluses that open up and start to bleed. My passion for bars made me the queen of rips. I taped them up and told myself to forget the pain for those few minutes I was competing. My feet hit the mat after my dismount and that was it, I was done. I had hit four for four and only had to wait to hear the results now!

The waiting time felt so long, but I knew I had done my personal best and that was enough to make me feel like the happiest girl in the world. My all around score was a 36.975. I couldn't believe I had increased that much.

We went to awards, and as they were announcing the floor awards they started at the bottom scores and moved to the top. They kept moving up and I thought to myself that there wasn't any way I took first. Surprising myself completely, I had taken first! They called my name and I wanted to cry I was so happy. I did it; I had surpassed the negative thoughts in my head and taken first place at a National Tournament. I felt unstoppable.

13

A HARD TIME

Immediately after I competed at Nationals, I decided I had to tell someone about the back pain I had been dealing with during training for Nationals. I had been training so hard and taking care of my diabetes that I hadn't been taking care of my physical and emotional health very well. My Mom took me to the doctor and I had an X-Ray and an MRI done. Sure enough, I had fractured part of my lower vertebrae. At the time of my diagnosis I began to cry. I knew this would set me back, and more importantly, cause problems in my future gymnastics career. The next three months, all of summer, I had to wear a back brace and stop water skiing and gymnastics.

When summer was over my fracture had healed and it was time to start physical therapy. After a month of physical therapy, my therapist said I was strong enough to go back to gymnastics. I had to do strengthening and conditioning for at least a month before I would have half the strength I did before the fracture. It felt like I had lost it all...my skills, my strength, and my confidence. It felt like I was starting all over.

When I actually started getting back into my skills, it wasn't the same. I felt a constant back pain, and that is when I had to see a doctor at the Children's Hospital. My back had not only suffered from a fracture but I had mild disc degeneration, arthritis, and a bone that grew back thicker in the spot of the fracture. Ultimately, my doctor told me I had to be done with gymnastics. If I wanted to be able to continue to walk without pain when I was thirty I had to "retire."

At the moment my doctor gave me the news I burst into tears. Everything I had been working for was gone. I had spent 11 years in that gym, and practiced over 8,000 hours. It was all done, I couldn't believe it.

After that, I felt so stressed emotionally. I was dealing with depression from not only my loss of gymnastics, but also because my Dad had been dealing with some health problems (a diagnosis of cancer). On top of all that, I was struggling finding a friend to talk to about it all. As a result of my decreased level of activity I had to figure out completely new doses of insulin for all times of the day. Depending on the day and the weather and whether I was sad, happy, anxious, depressed—my blood sugar would do different things each day. I needed help, someone to talk to, someone to guide me about how to manage everything at once. I never asked my Mom, because I already knew the worry she went through for me. She worried about my health and safety every day, and I didn't want to add to her burden. My

Dad had health problems of his own that were much more important to deal with, and I wanted to make things easier on him, not harder. My sisters were busy with school work and their own lives, and because they were all at college, they no longer lived at home. Most of my friends, although kind, would not have known what to say. I didn't think they would understand what was going on in my life. I eventually found myself opening up about everything going on, and this is when my friends and family stepped up to help. How could I have expected them to know without telling them? I am private with my personal life, but opening up to people dearest to me was the best thing I had done.

At that time I wished I could have talked to another Type One that could have offered me advice and connected with me. This brings me to the reason I am writing this book, to give other people dealing with Type One Diabetes another story to understand what it's like, and a person to talk to if they need it. As I have learned, It is just as important to take care of your mental, emotional and physical health as it is your diabetes management.

14

MOVING FORWARD

THE YEAR of 2016-2017 was one of the hardest years I had gone through, but it made me much stronger physically and emotionally. The next year I knew I had to make my comeback year. I started to get back into working out intensely, though nothing like my gymnastics. I noticed my blood sugar levels were leveling out better like they did when I was in gymnastics. It was crazy how much happier I was when my blood sugars were normal.

Since I was no longer training gymnastics 16+ hours a week, I found myself with a lot of extra time I never had before. Gymnastics was a big stress reliever for me in the past, and missing that piece was continuing to make me depressed. I decided to get back into playing the piano. I learned how to play the ukulele and guitar also, and I even got a couple of jobs coaching gymnastics. These things helped me escape my worries and anxiety momentarily. Though nothing would compare to my love for gymnastics, these things felt like they saved me.

Everything looked a little bit brighter. I was more hopeful now. The summer of 2017 my doctor said I could waterski again. I had much more time to improve on my water skiing without practicing gymnastics, and I had set a new goal to ski in college. I had even received an opportunity to do doubles with a professional team in Japan, but sadly had to turn it down because I wasn't 18 yet. Receiving that invitation was enough to motivate me to get better and stronger that summer.

In this year of "moving forward" I was selected to participate in the Miss Wisconsin Teen USA competition. I was one of about 30 girls selected in the state of WI. At first I was hesitant because I didn't have much confidence in myself but I ended up doing the competition. I looked at it as a way to represent T1D and show that it was still possible to be beautiful with the chronic illness. It was completely out of my comfort zone and empowering. I hadn't expected to win any awards because most girls had prepared most of their lives for an opportunity like this. I had won the highest scoring formal gown award! This award meant so much more than a plaque to me. It showed me I still had confidence somewhere inside me. I learned I could still be unstoppable despite an unfortunate previous year.

This year of moving forward reminded me to not let the negatives affect my life. I am now a senior in high school. I have learned many things from the past 6 years having Type One Diabetes. From here on out, I will continue to never let Type One Diabetes stop me. When I have doubts, from myself or other people, I will look back at the things I have overcome and know nothing will stop me. Don't let T1D ever stop you.

15

***

JDRF

The Juvenile Diabetes Research Foundation (JDRF) has done remarkable things, and with all of our help they will continue to break down barriers and get closer to a cure.

When I was first diagnosed, Insulin pumps were still relatively new. Since then, I have seen many scientific discoveries unfold. This research includes: beta cells, prevention treatments, artificial pancreas, and more. It is truly remarkable what the future holds, and what is already here!

In the past few years, I have tried to become more involved with JDRF by attending research updates, galas, and volunteering in any way possible. I do this because what they have accomplished has changed my life in so many ways. If there is any way I can give back to JDRF, I am willing to do it.

I will be giving a speech at the 2019 JDRF Gala in February to help raise awareness and more fundraising. I hope to impact the world through my work with JDRF, and I know that by taking little steps I will get there.

FOR ALL PEOPLE WITH T1D

1. You are not alone.

Despite feelings of being "different" and isolated because of the daily responsibilities T1D brings, you are not alone. Look, you just met another Type One, me! No one should have to feel it is up to themselves to manage something as complex as T1D. There are different camps, support groups, and resources to come into contact with other Type One's. Sometimes the best way to get through a hard day is to talk to someone else that may be dealing with similar things. Though each Type One Diabetic has to manage their diabetes differently, depending on what their body needs, it can be helpful to talk to other people. Please contact me at jordynmarlysjones@gmail.com if you are looking for support and are having trouble finding it.

2. Bad days are okay.

Nobody has perfect days, and it is okay to have a bad day.

You are not going to be able to predict how every single food you eat, or how each activity you do is going to affect your blood sugar. That is why it is important to realize you can only do so much. Do not blame yourself for your bad days- you will find a way to get past it and start fresh the next day.

3. It is not your fault.

There is nothing you did or didn't do to give Type One Diabetes to yourself. Whether it be genetic or unknown, the cause of your Type One Diabetes couldn't have been prevented. Do not blame yourself.

4. So many things can affect your diabetes that are out of your control.

Yes, so very many things can affect your blood sugars in ways you may not even know. Things such as the weather, activity, stress, sleep, hormonal changes, and of course food. Realizing that most of these things are out of your control can be very frustrating. Dealing with out of range blood sugars when you don't know what is causing it can be very frustrating. Just breathe and realize you can't control everything. You and your doctor will manage the unexpected things as best as you can.

5. Your quality of life is the same.

Just because you have a "chronic illness" does not mean the quality of your life is going to change for the worse. Things may be more challenging with the responsibilities you have, but they are not impossible. If you set your mind to something, don't let your Type One Diabetes stop you from reaching that goal.

6. Don't be afraid to ask for help.

Again, you are not alone. Do not be afraid to ask a friend, a family member, or a doctor for help when you need it. With a diagnosis of Type One it can be overwhelming and confusing at first. You do not need to manage everything on your own. Reach out, even if it is for something as small as asking your friend to count the carbs when they are making you a batch of cookies. The smallest things like this help on days you feel overwhelmed.

7. Wear a medical ID bracelet.

I can not count the number of times my Mom has yelled at me for leaving the house without a medical ID bracelet on. I used to ignore the importance of what a medical bracelet would do for me until I realized it can mean the difference between life and death. Extreme hypoglycemia or hyperglycemia can lead to passing out, and if this unfortunate event were to happen when you are alone or with someone who is unaware that you have diabetes, it can be very dangerous. Wear a medical ID bracelet not only to save your life, but to put your loved ones at ease that you will be safe when you are not with them!

8. Don't be afraid to tell friends and family about your condition.

Everyday you will have risks of extreme high and low blood

sugars. Telling your closest friends and family about your T1D can be life saving. If they know how to watch for symptoms and how to act in emergencies, they can prevent dangerous situations from happening!

9. Spread Awareness whenever you can.

Trust me, I know it is not easy having Type One Diabetes in the world we live in today. Many people have false assumptions about the disease and do not understand what really causes it. Some assumptions even categorize Type One Diabetes and Type Two Diabetes into one disease, when in fact they are two completely different diseases. Each has different causes, and different forms of treatment. Spreading awareness of Type One Diabetes is the only way to educate people so they understand what it truly is. This doesn't mean you have to tell every single person you meet in your life, but if someone asks a question about that insulin pump you are wearing, just know that it can benefit you to answer in an honest and informative way.

FOR PEOPLE THAT KNOW SOMEONE
WITH T1D

1. Learn the effects of blood sugar levels.

As a friend or family member of someone dealing with Type One, it is important to know the symptoms of hyperglycemia and hypoglycemia. Becoming aware of these gives you the power to prevent dangerous situations and even save a life. This also means knowing where their glucagon is kept. This is absolutely life saving in hypoglycemia cases that result in passing out.

2. There are no food restrictions.

A common misconception with T1D is that we are not allowed to eat sugar. Yes we can eat whatever we want, we just need to know the proper amount of insulin to take so our blood sugars remain in the appropriate range. Occasionally, we may have to say no to a dessert if our blood sugar is high, but other than that we can manage to eat the foods we want.

3. Be aware of the causes of T1D.

A common misconception is that we caused this disease by eating too much sugar as a child, or being chubby as a child. NO. This disease is unpreventable (as of now) and we did not do anything to cause the disease. Though it commonly develops among people as children, it can happen to anyone at any age.

4. It does not restrict our abilities.

Having Type One Diabetes does not restrict our abilities to strive for our goals and be what we want to be. Yes, we may need to take more precautions for our health and safety, but it does not put up a barrier to reach our goals.

5. Don't be afraid to offer help.

Though we may seem to have everything "under control" the truth is that we can use help sometimes. Even in the smallest ways, maybe counting the carbs of that dinner you made for them, or comforting them on a bad day can help make it a better day.

6. Be understanding.

Not every day is a good day. Anything and everything can affect blood sugar levels. When blood sugars are out of range it can cause fatigue, tiredness, and abnormal actions. Be understanding if they are not feeling/acting like themselves, because it is not their fault.

PHOTOS

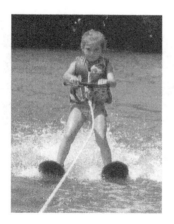

First learning how to ski at age four on Lake Miltona
in 2005

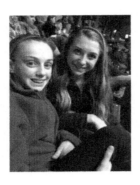

Gymnastics trip to Texas in January, 2013 (2 days prior to diagnosis)

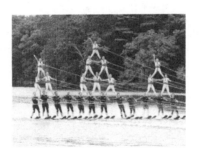

Skiing with Waterboard Warriors Waterski Team

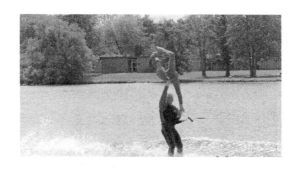

Waterski Doubles Nationals in 2013

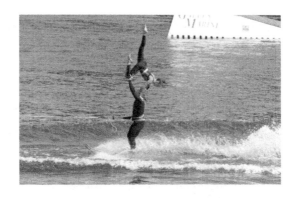

Waterski Doubles State in 2015

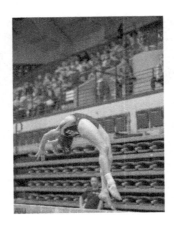

Level 9 Nationals in Missoula, Montana in 2016

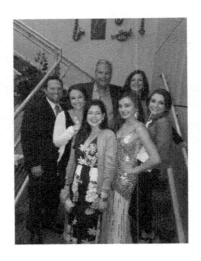

Family Picture at Miss WI Teen USA Competition in 2017

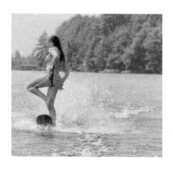

Waterskiing during the summer of 2018

CONTACT ME

Whether you have Type One Diabetes or are a friend to someone with Type One Diabetes, I hope my story will inspire you to live your best life. Remember, you are unstoppable, you are beautiful, and you are magnificent. Do not let T1D stop you. Let it inspire you to rise above and do amazing things. Rise above the doubt and fear, follow people that inspire you, and keep people in your life that support you. Please contact me if you or someone you know could use someone to talk to about their Type One Diabetes and the struggles that come with it.

Made in the USA
Monee, IL
11 March 2021

62385143R00039